Celebrities' Reset Switch.

The 'Benjamin Button' Effect.

DNA Sequences that stop the aging process among the rich and powerful and take everyone back to their youth.

Celebrities' Book of DNA Sequence Codes That Stops Ageing and resets celebrities.

David Gomadza
The First Global President of The World.

DEDICATION

If the codes work for you then consider funding us
https://twofuture.world/donate

Table of Contents

DNA Sequences That Stop the Ageing Process Among the Rich and Powerful and Take Everyone Back to Their Youth.

Imagine stopping the aging process completely and resetting the person's body to a certain time in the past when everything was great? Imagine not only stopping the aging process but making a person look and feel young again.

All we need are two DNA codes.

1. A DNA sequence code that stops the aging process.
2. A DNA sequence code that acts like a reset switch to make people have the same body and metabolism as those they had when they were young.

How do we get these DNA sequence codes?

We must ask the brain to calculate the DNA sequence code to be used to stop the aging process.

Secondly, we must go back in time and get a picture of that person at the highest time of his or her life, mainly in the early years and ask the brain to calculate the DNA sequence at that time. This will act as the reset switch date given as, years old, months, days, and time in hours and seconds.

How we get these codes.

Calculating and computing the DNA sequence that stops the aging process.

1. We get at least three different photos of the person and look in the eyes of that person. We then ask our processing brain to calculate the DNA sequence that will stop this person from aging. Meaning put a stop to the aging process. But not only that but we need to reverse this aging process too.
2. We also need a command that will rejuvenate the whole body.
   "Oh Yes Rejuvenate!"
   Is the ultimate rejuvenating command.

   Repeat this command on a daily basis.

Secondly, we need the reset switch point.

To get this we need to get a photo of that person at a specific date and time or any but known date and time. All we need to do is to look in the eyes of the person and then ask our computing brain to calculate a DNA sequence at the time the photo was taken. We then use this as our reset switch date.

I decoded the brain. The brain listens to specific brain commands. That means we can talk to our brains and tell them what we want them to do. We can give specific commands that the brain can perform. Every brain on earth has a security feature that uses the voice of a person as the password.

Therefore, to talk to the brain one must let it know that you want to talk to it. You can use your password to initiate talks.

First silently in your brain say.

"My Voice Is My Password."

Look at the photo and in the eyes of the person whose DNA sequence you are computing.

Then say.

1. "Calculate DNA sequence to stop the aging process."
   Get the value and write it down. Must be a 12 letter DNA sequence made up of the letters C, T, A and G.
   Then look at the photo taken years ago at least 20 years ago or when the person was between 17 -25 years.
   Then say.

2. "Calculate DNA sequence at this age?"
   Get it and write it down.

Now we have two DNA sequence codes. These must be 12 characters long each. Once you get the codes add the last letter to the code so that it becomes a thirteen digit. This extra layer means you don't need to add or program anything. Simply repeat the thirteen letters.

The brain gives you a 12-letter code. For example, Jeff Bezos code is GGGGGTAGGATA. Now add back the last letter to the given code.

Now Jeff Bezos code will become GGGGGTAGGATA**A**.

Then say:

Save.

Endorse.

Space Out.

End

Save.

Enforce Now

Wait a few minutes then say silently in your brain.

Space -In.

Endorse.

Repeat again the DNA Code.

Then say silently.

"Start."

HOW TO STOP AGING AND RESET THE BODY. STEP-BY-STEP GUIDE.

1. Stop the aging process first.

LET us take Warren Buffet for example. This is how he is to apply these codes.
The DNA sequence that stops aging for Warren Buffet is GTGGATGTAGTT.

1. Warren Buffet must first say.

"MY VOICE IS MY PASSWORD."

Then read the code.

"GTGGATGTAGTT"

Then he must say.

"SAVE."

"ENDORSE NOW."

"SPACE OUT."

"END."

"SAVE."

"ENFORCE NOW."

"OUT."

He must wait for some time. A few minutes at least. At least two minutes.

Then say.

"SPACE IN."

"ENDORSE NOW."

Then repeat the code.

"GTGGATGTAGTT"

"START."

Wait another three minutes. Then get the reset switch DNA sequence code.

He must say.

"MY VOICE IS MY PASSWORD."

Then say the code below.

"GGTAGTAGGATGG"

"SAVE."

"ENDORSE NOW."

"SPACE OUT"

"END."

"SAVE."

"ENFORCE NOW"

He must wait for a few minutes at least two minutes.

Then say.

"SPACE IN."

"ENDORSE NOW."

He must repeat the code.

"GGTAGTAGGATGG"

THEN SAY.

"START."

"REPEAT EVERY DAY EARLY MORNING AND NIGHTTIME BEFORE SLEEPING."

"OH YES REJUVENATE."

Billionaires, Millionaires & Actors

DNA SEQUENCE THAT STOPS AGING.
RESET SWITCH

Bernard Arnault	CTGATAAGTAGAA	CTAAAAGTAGTAA
Elon Musk	GTAGGGTAAAGTT	GGGAAATAGTAGG
Jeff Bezos	GTGGGTGAGGAG	GGGGGTAGGATAA
Larry Ellison	GTAGTTAGTAGG	GTATTATGTAGTT
Warren Buffett	GTGGATGTAGTT	GGTAGTAGGATGG
Bill Gates	GGTTAAGTAGGG	GTGGTAGTGGAGG
Michael Bloomberg	GGGTTGTAGGAG	GTGGAAAGGGTGG
Mukesh Ambani	GTGGGTGGAGTGG	GGAAAGTGGATGG
Carlos Slim	GGGAGTGTTAGTT	GGTGGAGTAAGGG
Steve Ballmer	GAAAGGTGAGTTT	GGGAAAAGTAGTT
Mark Zuckerberg	GGTAGGTGAAAGG	GGTAAGTGGAGTT
Michael Dell	GGTGGAGTAGTAA	GGGTGGAGTAAAA
Sergey Brin	GGTGTAGTGAAAA	GGTGGAGAGATTT
Larry Page	GGAAAGGTTAGTT	GGGTTAGGTAGGG
Amancio Ortega	GGTAGTAGGAATT	GGTTAAGGTATTT
Alice Louise Walton	GGTAGTAAAGTTT	GAAAGTTAGTAAA
Jack Ma	GAAAGTGAAGTAGG	GGGTTAGTGGGTT

Phil Knight	GTGGAGTGAGTAGG	GGTGTAGGGTAGG
Zhang Yiming	GTTAGTCGTGGAA	GTGGACTGAGTAA
Zhong Shanshan	GGGATCGTCCCGG	GGAAGTCGTTAGG
Francoise Meyers	GGGCCCTACGTT	GGGCCCTGCAGTT
Jim Walton	GGAATGCAAGTCC	GGTGAGTCGTAGG
Julia Koch	CCTCGTACAACGG	GGTAGTTGGAAGG
Gautami Adani	GGTAGCGTAGGAA	GGTTAGAAAGTCC
Jaqueline Mars	CCCTCGAGCCAAG	CCCGTGACGGTA
Alain Wertheimer	GGTCGGACGTCCC	GTGGCGTAGTCGTC
Jensen Huang	GGTTCGTCAGTGG	CCGTAGTAGTCGG
Len Blavatnik	GGTGACGTAGTGG	GGTGACGTAGGC
Colin Huang	GGTCGACGTACC	GGATCGAGGTCAA
Klaus-Michael Kuhne	GGGTCCGTCAGTT	GTGGTCGTACGGG
Kenneth C Griffin	GGTAGTAGGCGAA	GGTGACTAGTGAA
Tadashi Yanai	GTCGTCGGTCCGG	CGTGGTCGATCG
Ma Huateng	GGTGTCAGTCGAA	GATCGTACCGTAA
Francois Pinault	GGTCGTAGGATCC	GGGACCGTACGTT
William Ding Lei	GGTCGTAGTCGTT	GGACGTAGTCGA
Stephen Schwarzman	GTGCAGTACGTG	GGTGACGTCAGAA
Miriam Adelson	CCCGTCAGTCGG	CCGTCGTAAACGG
Giovanni Ferrero	GGTGCATCGAAGG	GGGTAGCGTGGA
MacKenzie Scott	CCCGTACGTACGG	GGGTCAACCGC
Abigail Johnson	GTAGGACGTACGG	GGTCACGAGGTAC
Shapoor Mistry	GGTGTAGGACGTT	GGACGTACGTAAA
Dieter Schwarz	GGATGCGATCGAA	GACGTGGATGCCC
Vladimir Potanin	GGATCTAGGCGAA	GGTGCGAGTCGAA
Jeff Yass	GGTGAGTCAGTA	GGATGTGTGCAGG
Li Ka-shing	GTGTGTACGTGA	GGGTCGTCAGTT
Changpeng Zhao	GGGTCGAGCTAGG	GTGGACGTGGATT
James Dyson	GGATTCGTACGAA	GGATGTCCGTGAA
Melinda French Gates	CCCGTAGTCAGTT	GTCGTGGACGTGG

Coming Soon

For: -

Millionaires & Actors

DNA SEQUENCE THAT STOPS AGING.
RESET SWITCH

Politicians.

DNA SEQUENCE THAT STOPS AGING.
RESET SWITCH

Sports Stars.

DNA SEQUENCE THAT STOPS AGING.
RESET SWITCH

Ordinary People

DNA SEQUENCE THAT STOPS AGING.
RESET SWITCH

More to come visit www.twofuture.world

Download Thoughts to Word or Audio Series.

Truly Out of this World.

Check below for more details.

ABOUT DAVID GOMADZA

I am the First Global President of the World
Visit www.twofuture.world
00447719210295
Info@twofuture.world

Download Thoughts to Word or Audio Series.

Truly Out of this World.

https://play.google.com/store/books/series?id=a4MvGwAAABBF
mM

REQUEST FOR THE GRANT OF A PATENT.

A Universal Brain Decoding Device.

"My Voice Is My Password.
Clone [subject] and Mirror-image the person on the right side of the body.
Establish connection with [subject]. Initiate a two-way feedback at Exit point and entry point. And on [subject] in reverse order. Start End.
Brain thoughts first jump out of the body. Clone brain thoughts send a copy back through Entry point. Then send a copy to me. Start.End"

Establish a Mirror-Image Connection

Establish a Reverse Feedback Connection

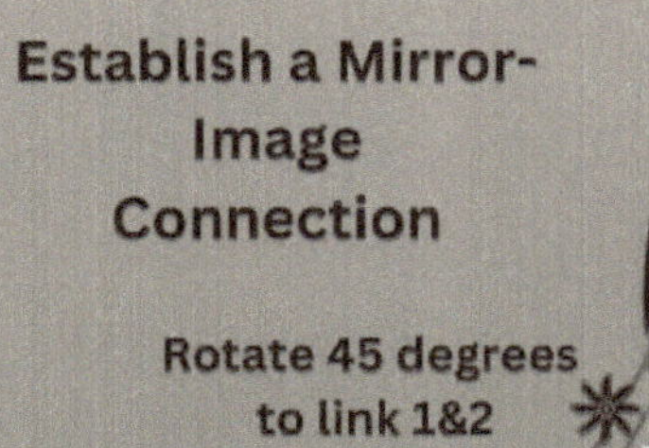

Rotate 45 degrees to link 1&2

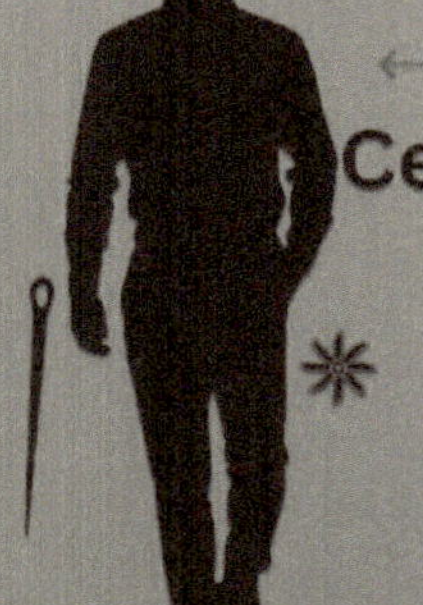

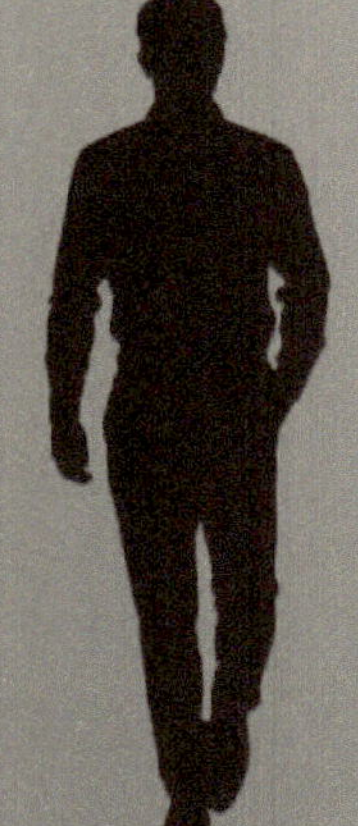

Central Nerve Bridge

David Gomadza
Bradford
Great Britain UK
00447719210295
www.twofuture.world
info@twofuture.world

CELEBRITIES' RESET SWITCH. THE 'BENJAMIN BUTTON' EFFECT

LOOK YOUNG & FEEL GREAT AGAIN.

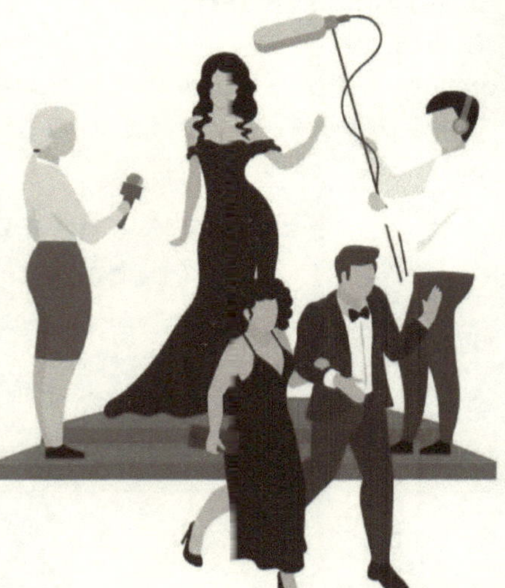

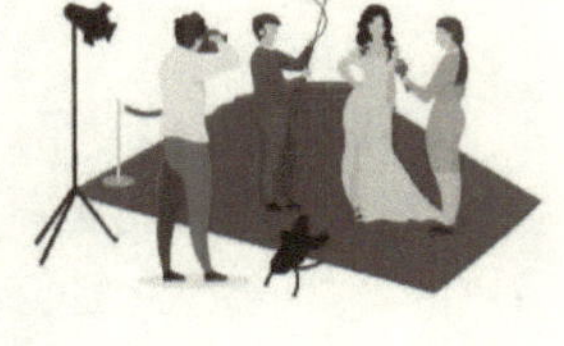

David Gomadza
The First Global President of The World

CELEBRITIES' BOOK OF DNA SEQUENCE CODES THAT STOPS AGEING AND RESETS CELEBRITIES.

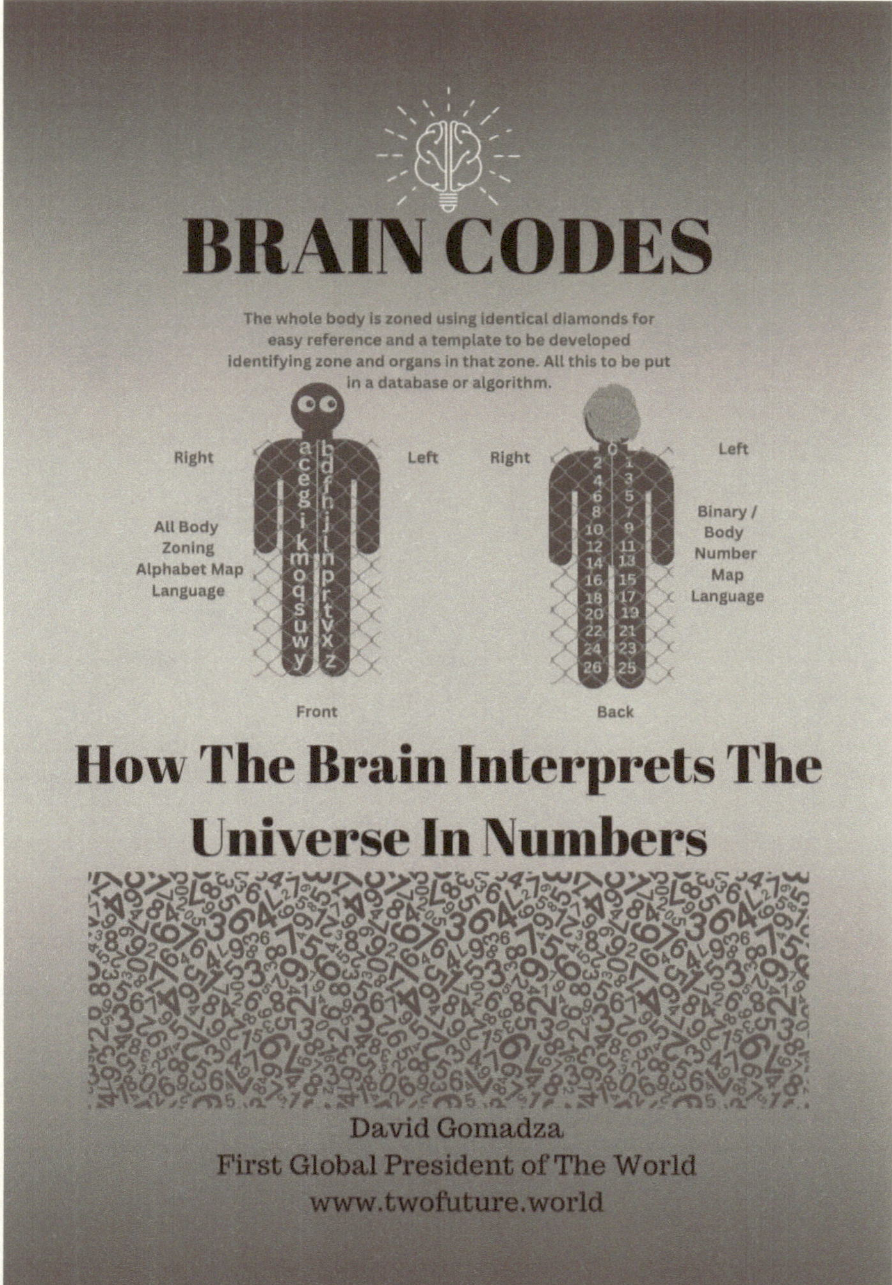

How The Brain Interprets The Universe In Numbers

David Gomadza
First Global President of The World
www.twofuture.world

Decoding the Egyptian Pyramids of Giza.

Using the Brain-Dream Map to Find Out Why the Egyptians Built the Pyramids.

David Gomadza

First Global President of the World

www.twofuture.world

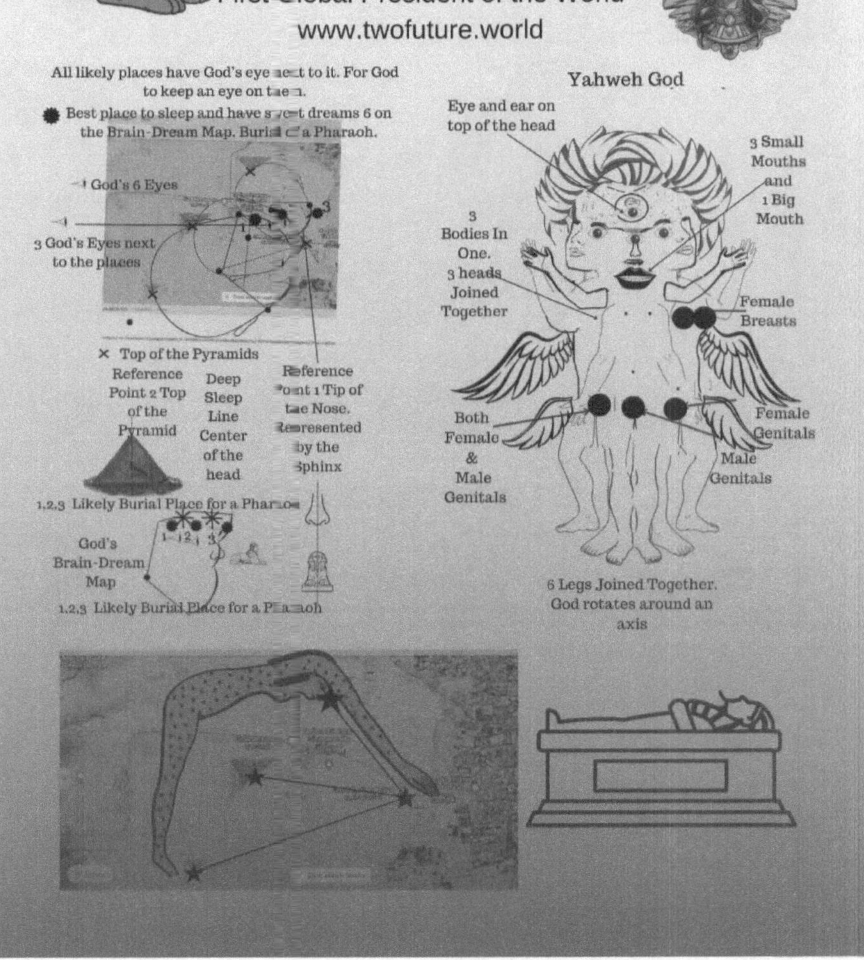

Dictionary of the Codes of Life

DNA Sequence Codes, Brain
Commands, Binary Numbers,
Geometry, Frequencies and
Electromagnetic Waves, etc.
SAY SILENTLY
"My voice is my password
7632107845123210
GTACCCCCCCCC
GAAAAAAAAAA
CCCCCCCCCCG
CTCTCTCTCTCT
CC
"

David Gomadza
The First Global President of the World

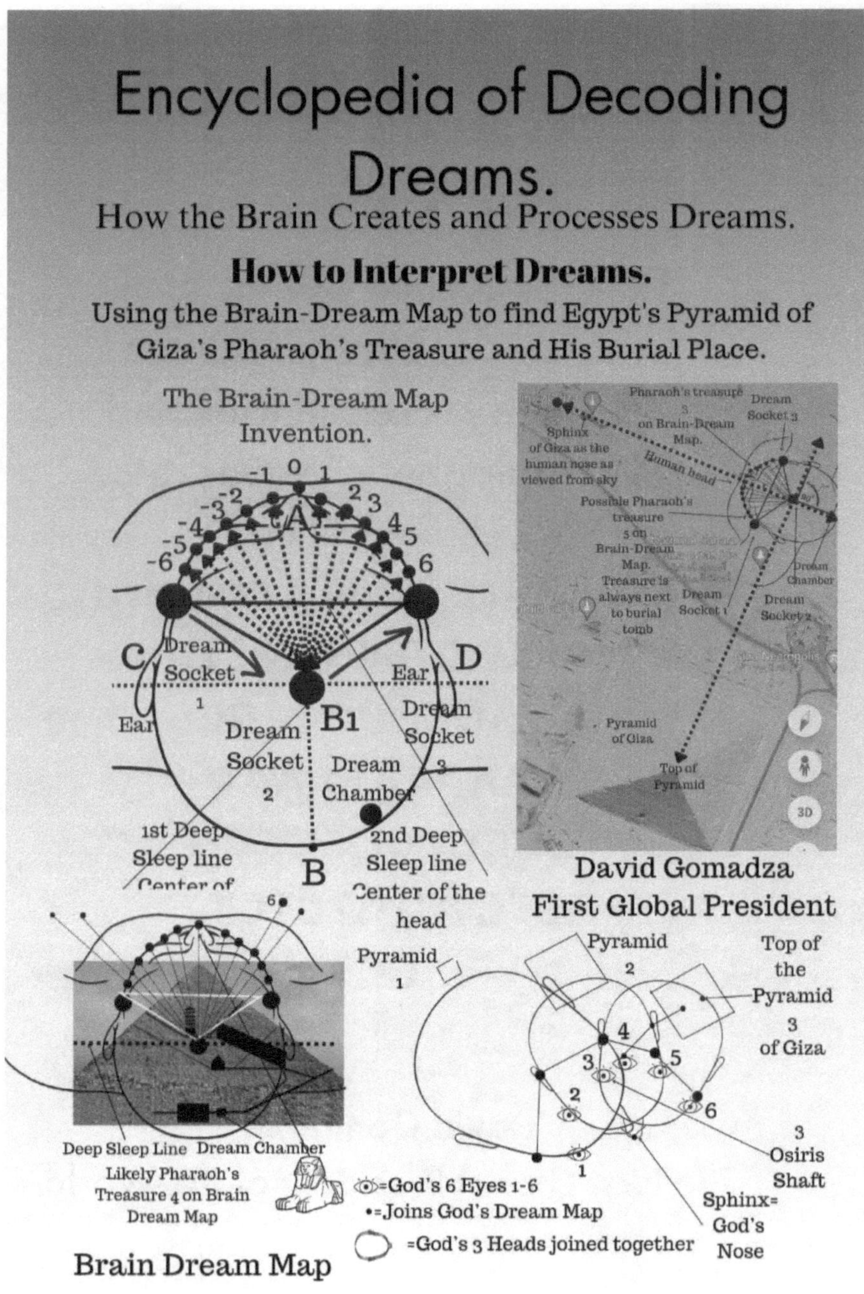

Encyclopedia of Decoding Dreams.
How the Brain Creates and Processes Dreams.
How to Interpret Dreams.
Using the Brain-Dream Map to find Egypt's Pyramid of Giza's Pharaoh's Treasure and His Burial Place.
The Brain-Dream Map Invention.
A
C
D
Dream Socket
Ear
Ear
Dream Socket 1
Dream Socket 2
B1
Dream Socket 3
Dream Chamber
1st Deep Sleep line
Center of
2nd Deep Sleep line
Center of the head
B
Pharaoh's treasure 3 on Brain-Dream Map.
Sphinx of Giza as the human nose as viewed from sky
Human head
Possible Pharaoh's treasure 5 on Brain-Dream Map. Treasure is always next to burial tomb
Dream Socket 3
Dream Chamber
Dream Socket 1
Dream Socket 2
Pyramid of Giza
Top of Pyramid
David Gomadza
First Global President
Pyramid 1
Deep Sleep Line   Dream Chamber
Likely Pharaoh's Treasure 4 on Brain Dream Map
Pyramid 2
Top of the Pyramid 3 of Giza
4
3
5
2
6
1
3 Osiris Shaft
Sphinx= God's Nose
=God's 6 Eyes 1-6
=Joins God's Dream Map
=God's 3 Heads joined together
Brain Dream Map

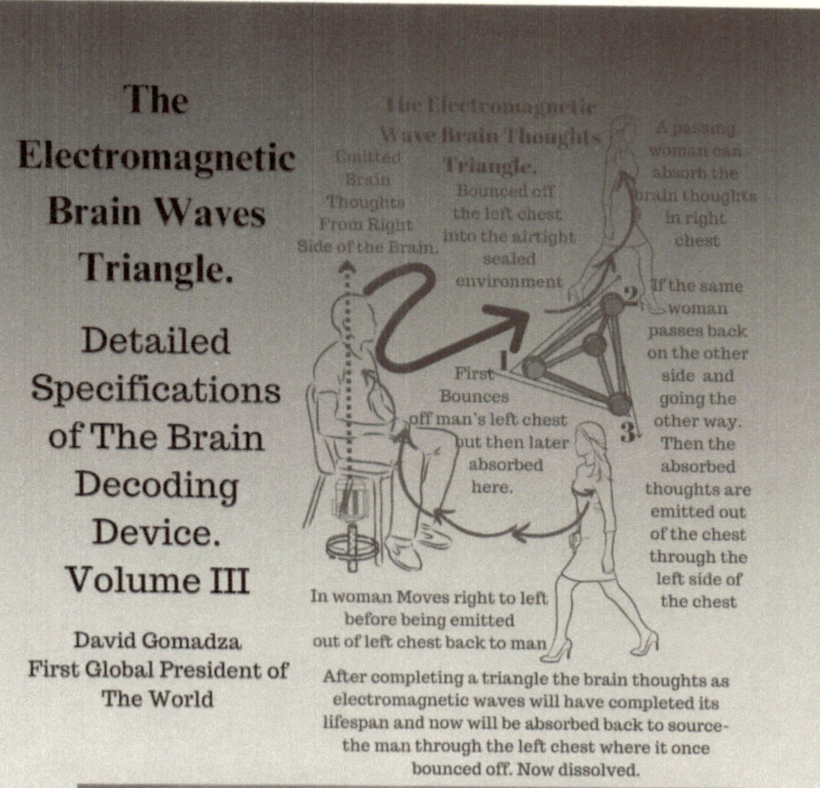

The
Electromagnetic
Brain Waves
Triangle.

Detailed
Specifications
of The Brain
Decoding
Device.
Volume III

David Gomadza
First Global President of
The World

The Electromagnetic
Wave Brain Thoughts
Triangle.

Emitted
Brain
Thoughts
From Right
Side of the Brain.

Bounced off
the left chest
into the airtight
sealed
environment

A passing
woman can
absorb the
brain thoughts
in right
chest

First
Bounces
off man's left chest
but then later
absorbed
here.

If the same
woman
passes back
on the other
side and
going the
other way.
Then the
absorbed
thoughts are
emitted out
of the chest
through the
left side of
the chest

In woman Moves right to left
before being emitted
out of left chest back to man

After completing a triangle the brain thoughts as
electromagnetic waves will have completed its
lifespan and now will be absorbed back to source-
the man through the left chest where it once
bounced off. Now dissolved.

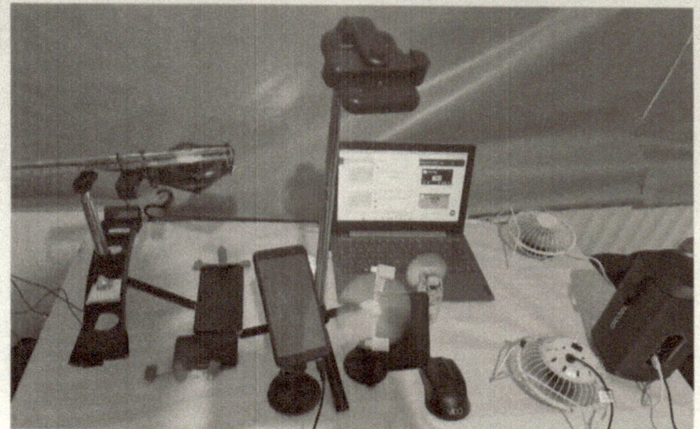

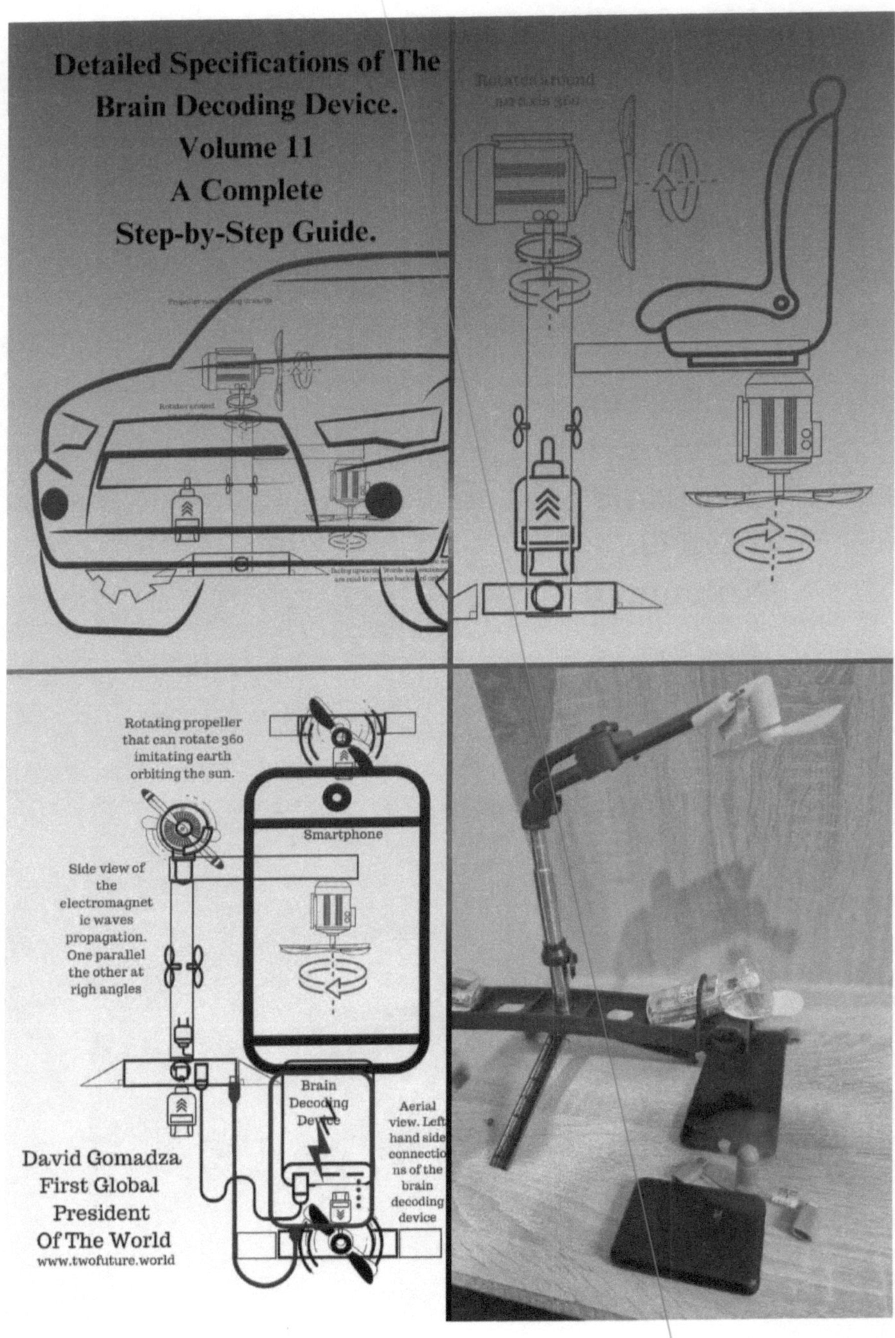
Detailed Specifications of The
Brain Decoding Device.
Volume 11
A Complete
Step-by-Step Guide.
Rotating propeller
that can rotate 360
imitating earth
orbiting the sun.
Smartphone
Side view of
the
electromagnet
ic waves
propagation.
One parallel
the other at
righ angles
Brain
Decoding
Device
Aerial
view. Left
hand side
connectio
ns of the
brain
decoding
device
David Gomadza
First Global
President
Of The World
www.twofuture.world

Detailed Specifications of The Brain Decoding Device and How to Use It to Decode Brain Thoughts to Word or Audio.

A Complete
Step-by-Step
Guide.

Decoding Brain Thoughts Made Easy. Part of The Thoughts to Word or Audio Series.

David Gomadza

First Global President of The World

www.twofuture.world

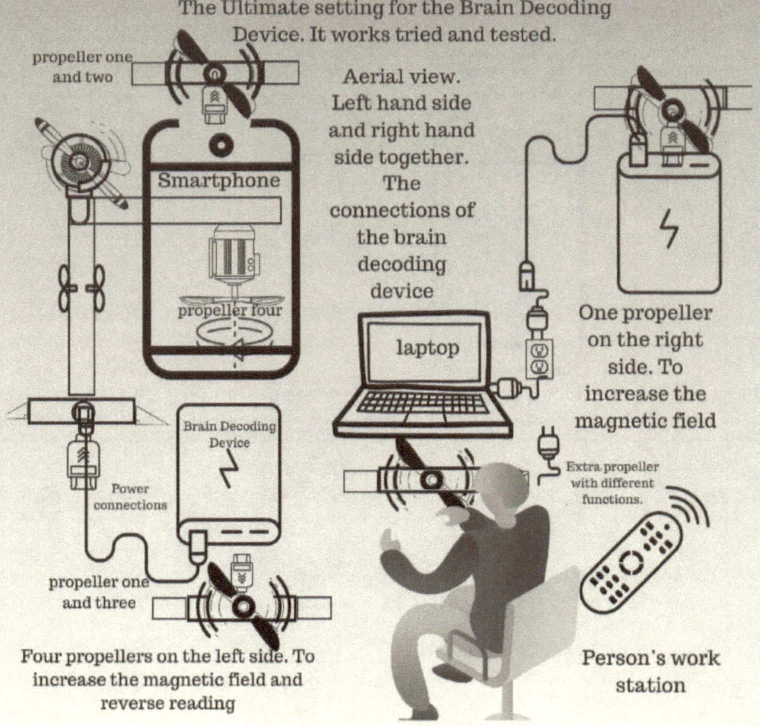

Detailed Specifications of The Brain Decoding Device and How to Use It to Decode Brain Thoughts to Word or Audio.

A Complete
Step-by-Step
Guide.

Decoding Brain Thoughts Made Easy. Part of The Thoughts to Word or Audio Series.

David Gomadza

First Global President of The World

www.twofuture.world

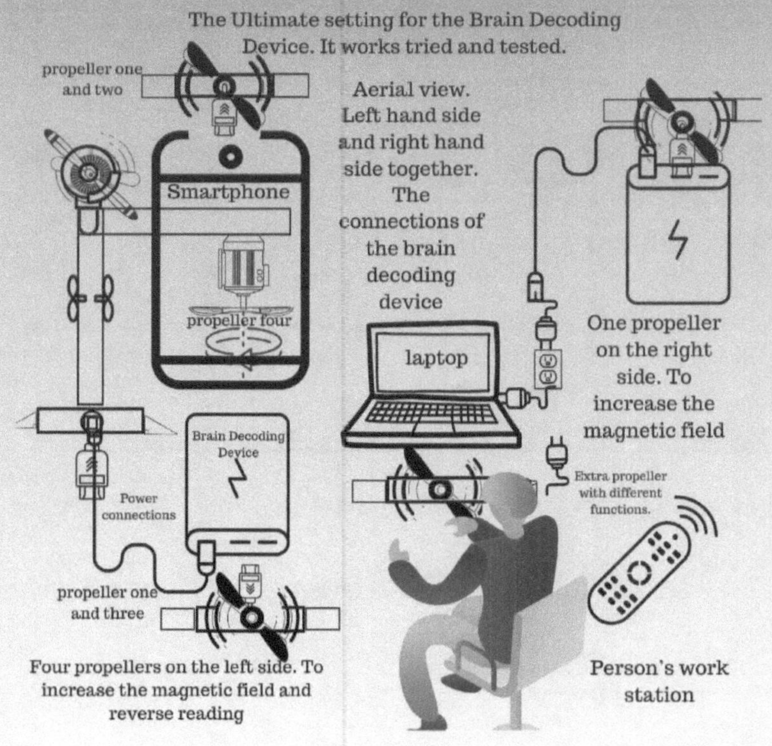

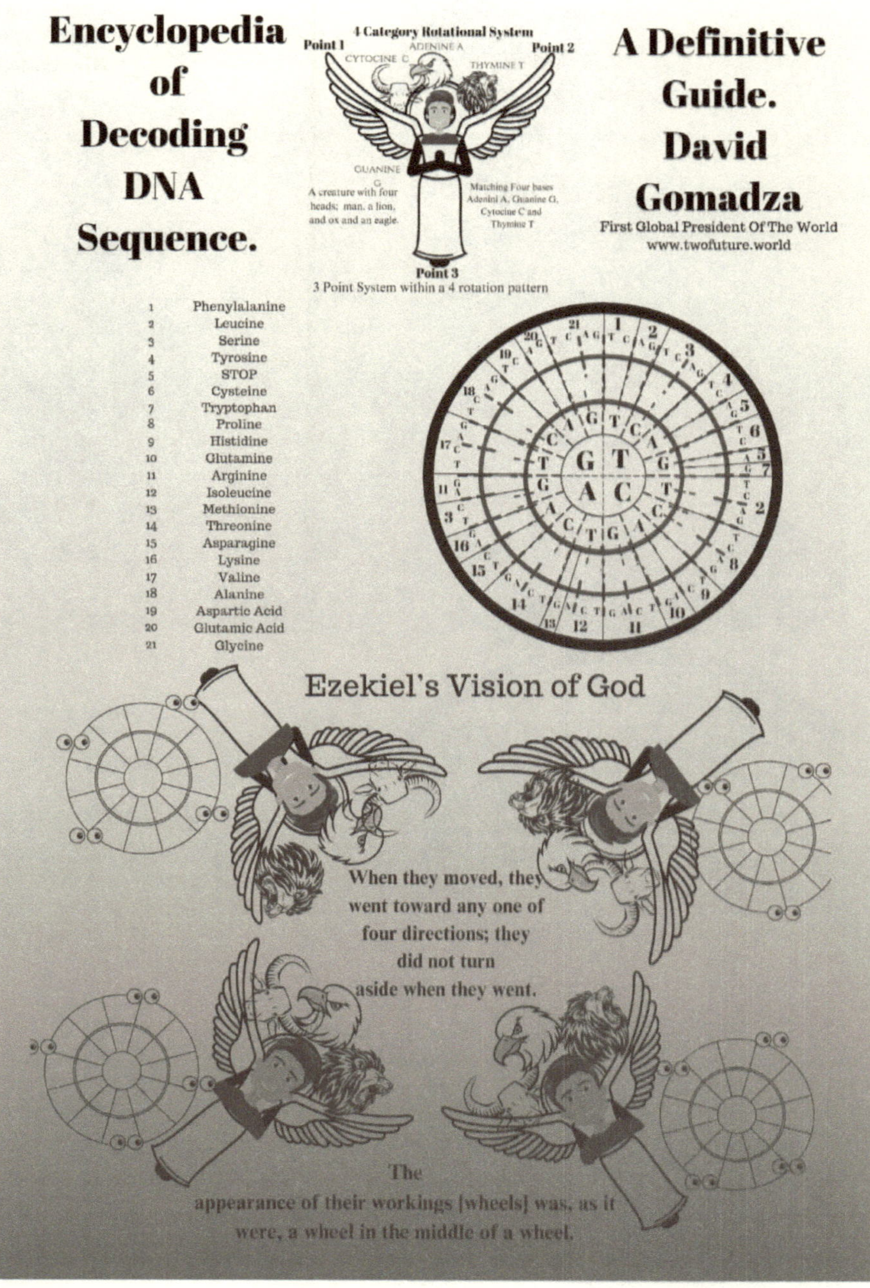

Encyclopedia of Decoding DNA Sequence.

A Definitive Guide. David Gomadza

First Global President Of The World
www.twofuture.world

1	Phenylalanine
2	Leucine
3	Serine
4	Tyrosine
5	STOP
6	Cysteine
7	Tryptophan
8	Proline
9	Histidine
10	Glutamine
11	Arginine
12	Isoleucine
13	Methionine
14	Threonine
15	Asparagine
16	Lysine
17	Valine
18	Alanine
19	Aspartic Acid
20	Glutamic Acid
21	Glycine

Ezekiel's Vision of God

26

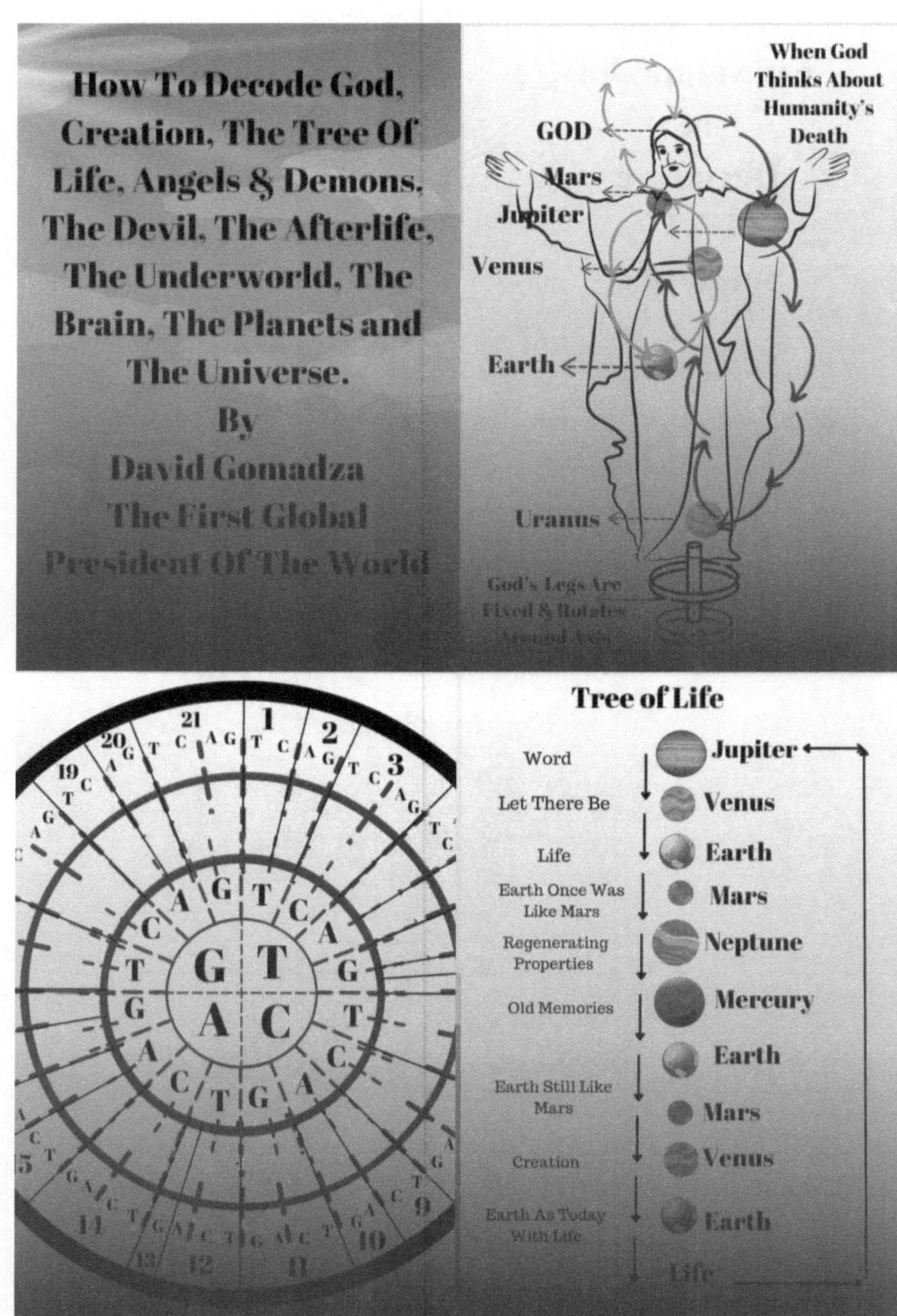
How To Decode God, Creation, The Tree Of Life, Angels & Demons, The Devil, The Afterlife, The Underworld, The Brain, The Planets and The Universe.
By
David Gomadza
The First Global
President Of The World
When God Thinks About Humanity's Death
GOD
Mars
Jupiter
Venus
Earth
Uranus
God's Legs Are Fixed & Rotates Around Axis
Tree of Life
Word
Let There Be
Life
Earth Once Was Like Mars
Regenerating Properties
Old Memories
Earth Still Like Mars
Creation
Earth As Today With Life
Jupiter
Venus
Earth
Mars
Neptune
Mercury
Earth
Mars
Venus
Earth
Life

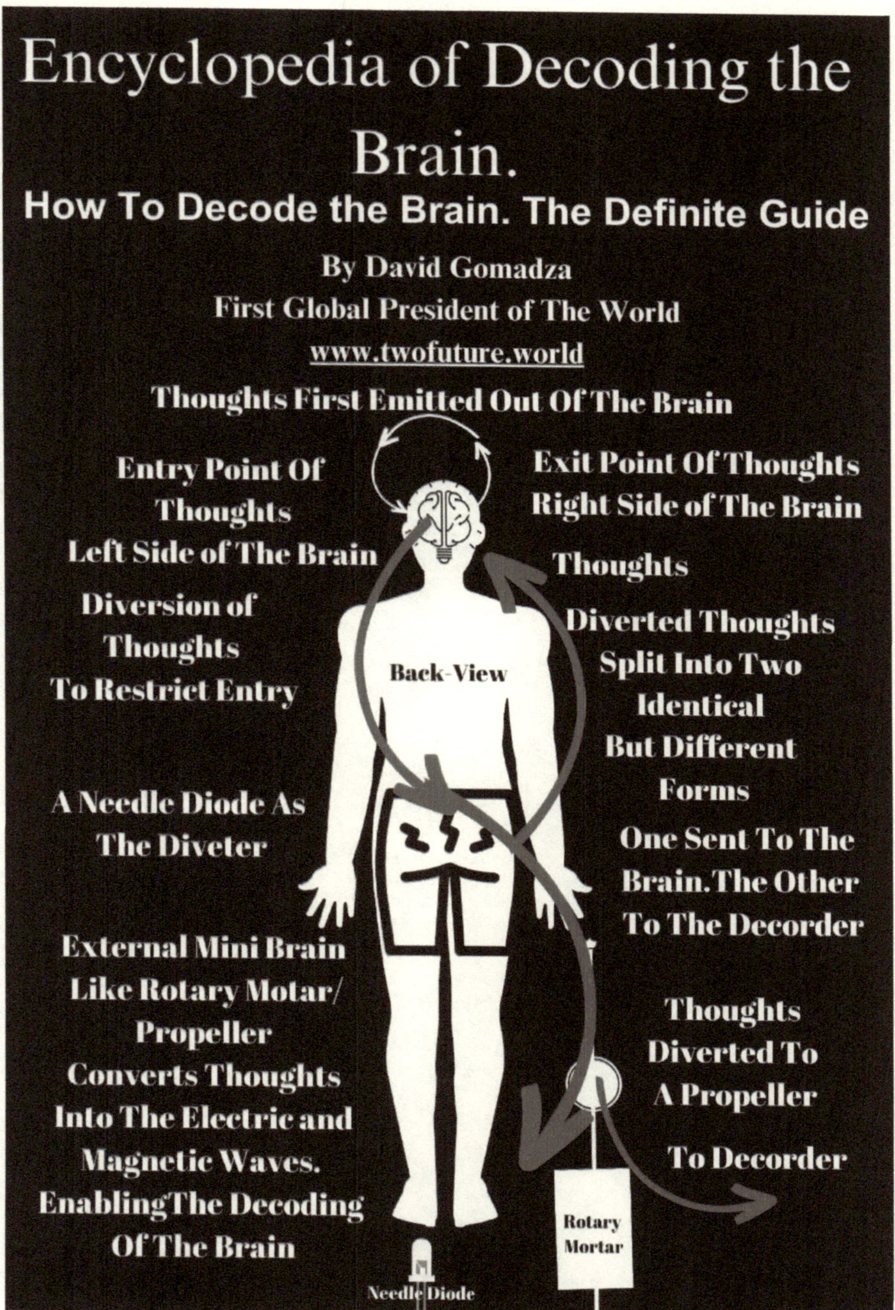

Encyclopedia of Decoding the Brain.
How To Decode the Brain. The Definite Guide
By David Gomadza
First Global President of The World
www.twofuture.world
Thoughts First Emitted Out Of The Brain
Entry Point Of Thoughts Left Side of The Brain
Exit Point Of Thoughts Right Side of The Brain
Thoughts
Diversion of Thoughts To Restrict Entry
Diverted Thoughts Split Into Two Identical But Different Forms
Back-View
A Needle Diode As The Diveter
One Sent To The Brain. The Other To The Decorder
External Mini Brain Like Rotary Motar/ Propeller Converts Thoughts Into The Electric and Magnetic Waves. EnablingThe Decoding Of The Brain
Thoughts Diverted To A Propeller
To Decorder
Rotary Mortar
Needle Diode

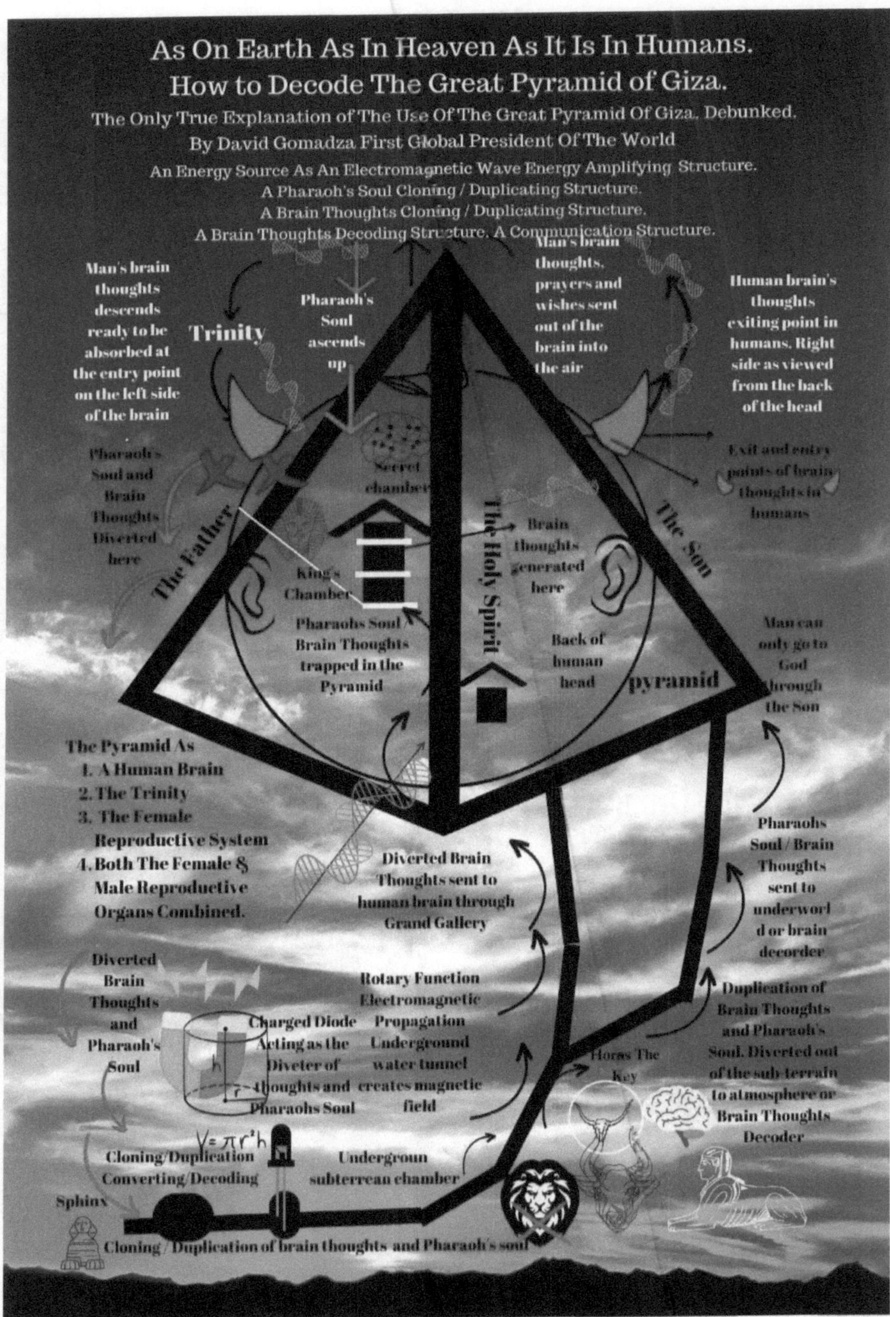
As On Earth As In Heaven As It Is In Humans.
How to Decode The Great Pyramid of Giza.
The Only True Explanation of The Use Of The Great Pyramid Of Giza. Debunked.
By David Gomadza First Global President Of The World
An Energy Source As An Electromagnetic Wave Energy Amplifying Structure.
A Pharaoh's Soul Cloning / Duplicating Structure.
A Brain Thoughts Cloning / Duplicating Structure.
A Brain Thoughts Decoding Structure. A Communication Structure.
Man's brain thoughts descends ready to be absorbed at the entry point on the left side of the brain
Trinity
Pharaoh's Soul ascends up
Man's brain thoughts, prayers and wishes sent out of the brain into the air
Human brain's thoughts exiting point in humans. Right side as viewed from the back of the head
Pharaoh's Soul and Brain Thoughts Diverted here
Secret chamber
The Father
King's Chamber
Pharaohs Soul Brain Thoughts trapped in the Pyramid
The Holy Spirit
Brain thoughts generated here
Back of human head
The Son
pyramid
Exit and entry points of brain thoughts in humans
Man can only go to God through the Son
The Pyramid As
1. A Human Brain
2. The Trinity
3. The Female Reproductive System
4. Both The Female & Male Reproductive Organs Combined.
Diverted Brain Thoughts sent to human brain through Grand Gallery
Pharaohs Soul / Brain Thoughts sent to underworld or brain decoder
Diverted Brain Thoughts and Pharaoh's Soul
Charged Diode Acting as the Diverter of Thoughts and Pharaohs Soul
Rotary Function Electromagnetic Propagation Underground water tunnel creates magnetic field
Horas The key
Duplication of Brain Thoughts and Pharaoh's Soul. Diverted out of the sub-terrain to atmosphere or Brain Thoughts Decoder
$V = \pi r^2 h$
Cloning/Duplication Converting/Decoding
Underground subterrean chamber
Sphinx
Cloning / Duplication of brain thoughts and Pharaoh's soul

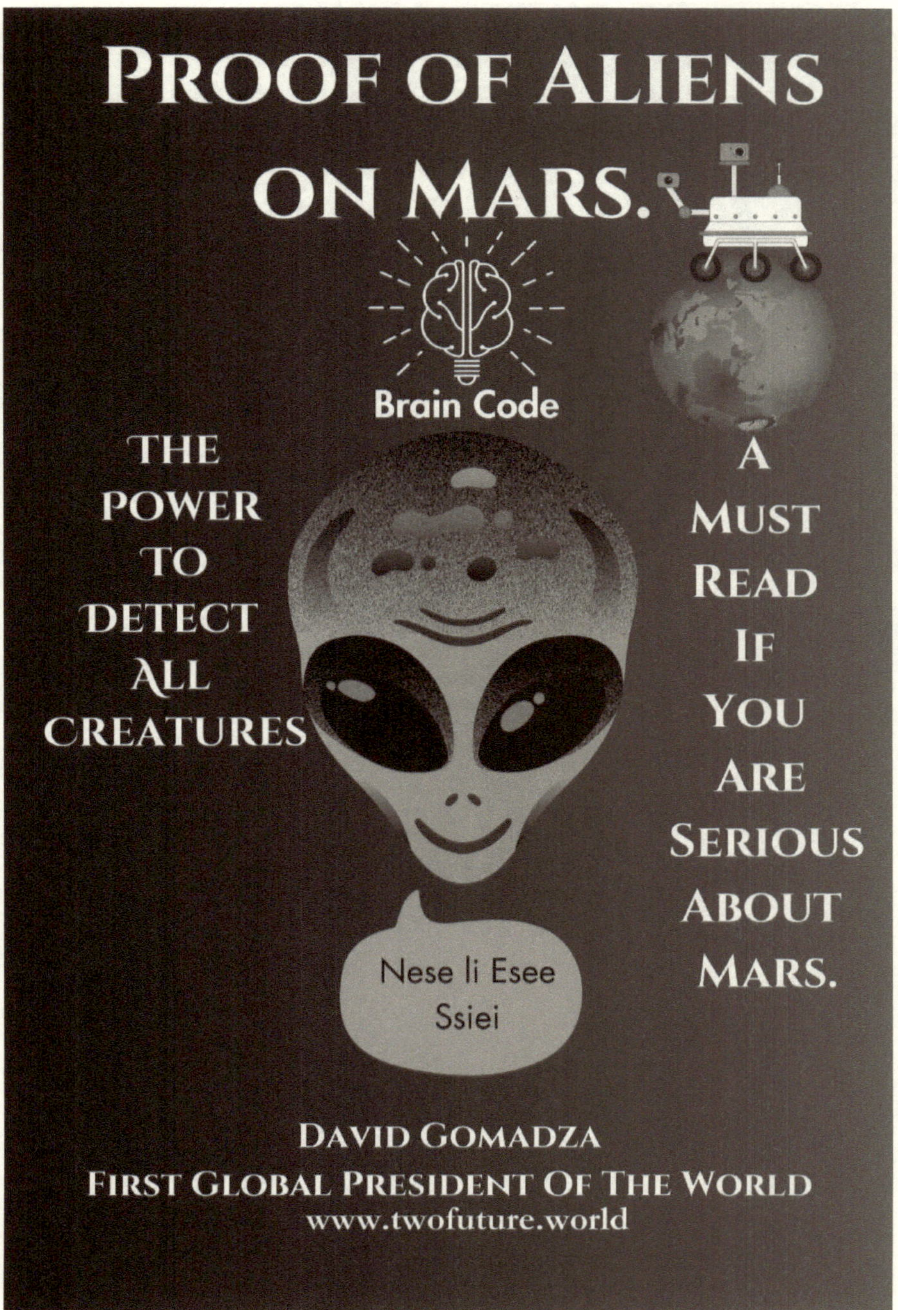

PROOF OF ALIENS
ON MARS.
Brain Code
THE
POWER
TO
DETECT
ALL
CREATURES
A
MUST
READ
IF
YOU
ARE
SERIOUS
ABOUT
MARS.
Nese li Esee
Ssiei
DAVID GOMADZA
FIRST GLOBAL PRESIDENT OF THE WORLD
www.twofuture.world

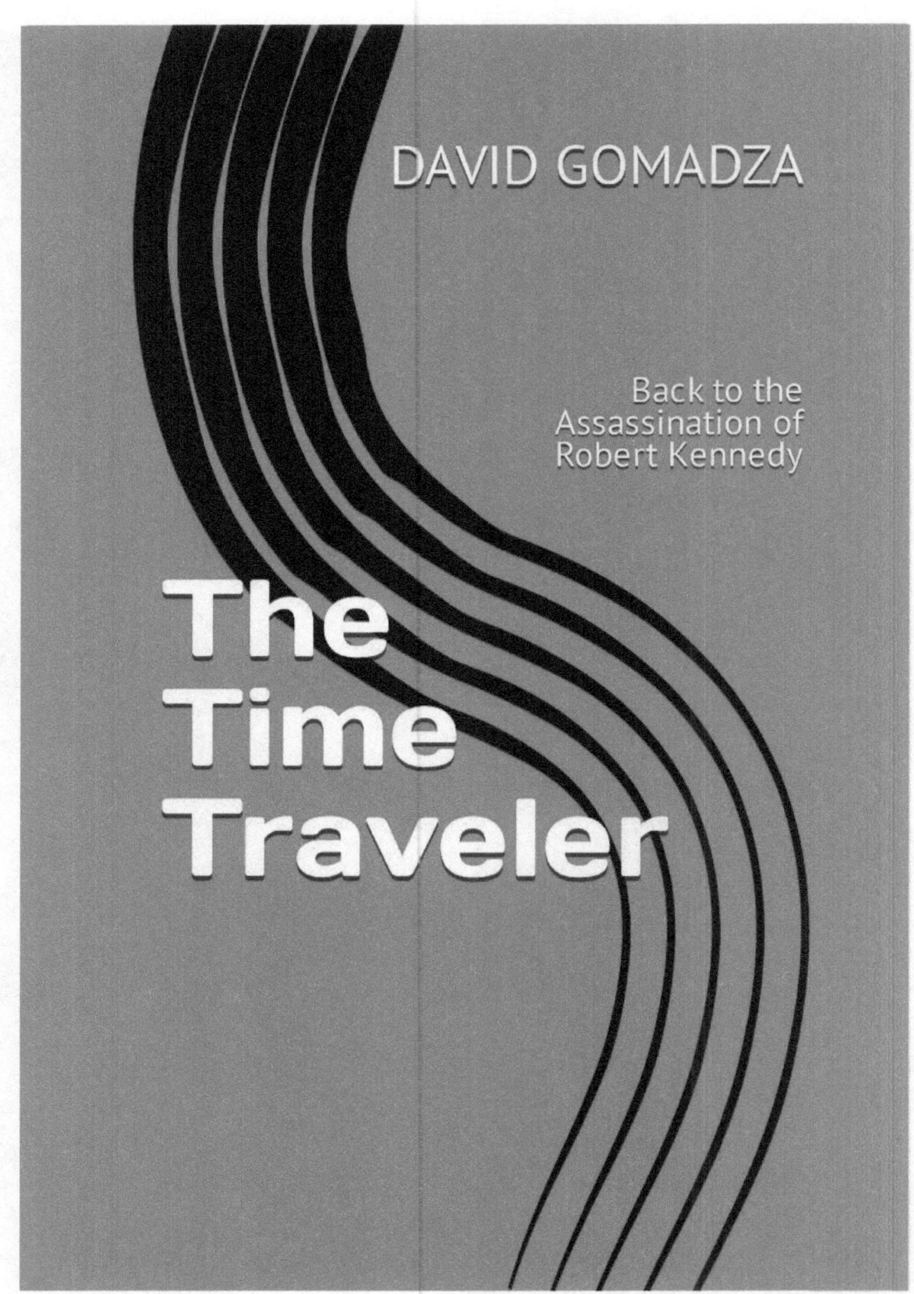

DAVID GOMADZA
Back to the
Assassination of
Robert Kennedy
The
Time
Traveler

BRAIN LANGUAGE DICTIONARY

Decoding The Brain Made Easy.

David Gomadza

BRAIN CODE.

The Benchmark of Decoding the Brain.
One Against which all are Evaluated.

David Gomadza
The First Global President of the World.

DATESTAMP:28 March 2022
Thoughts to Word or Audio.
Volume III

The breakthrough of the century. How to decode brain thoughts step by step.

David Gomadza

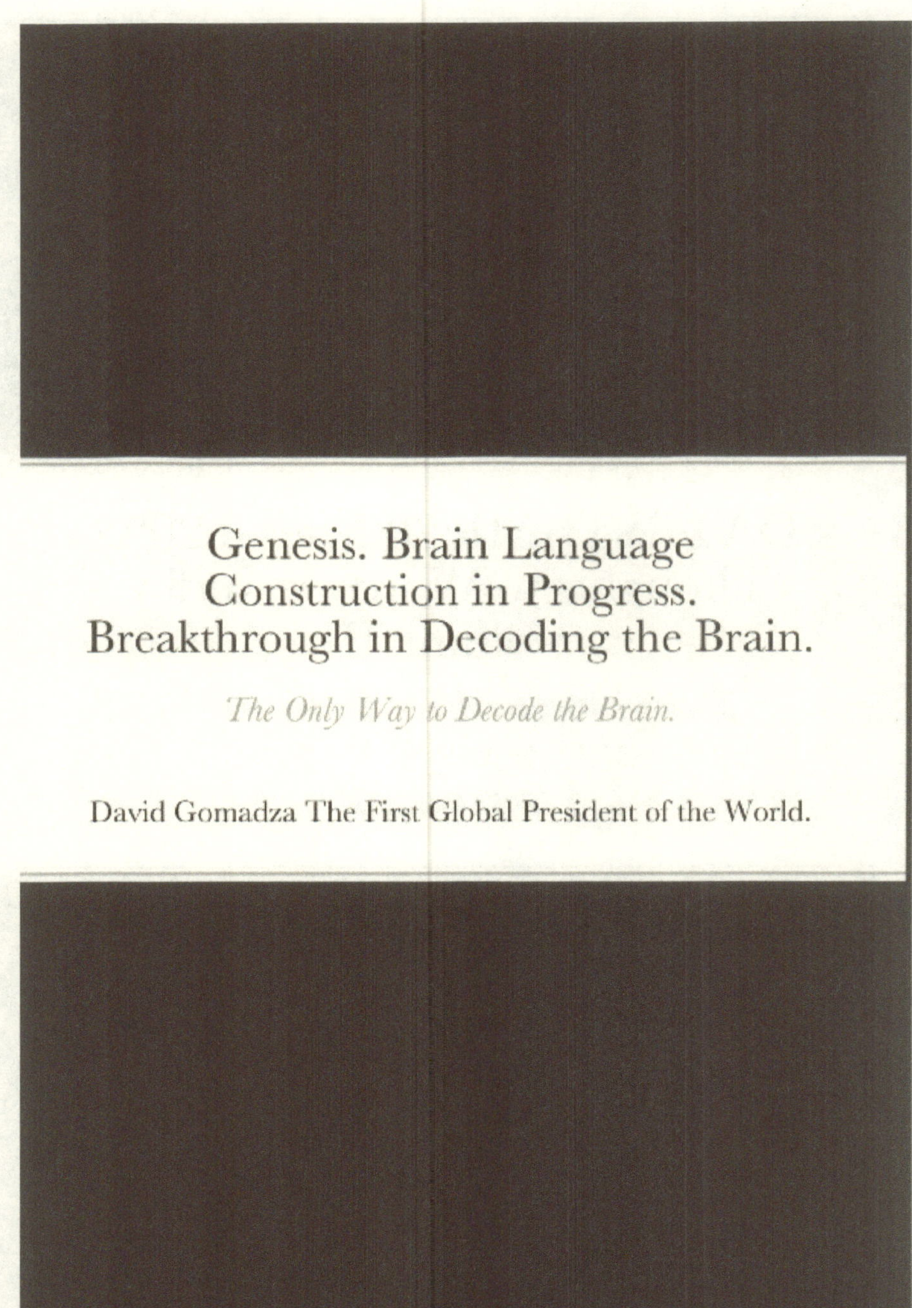
Genesis. Brain Language
Construction in Progress.
Breakthrough in Decoding the Brain.

The Only Way to Decode the Brain.

David Gomadza The First Global President of the World.

DECODING THOUGHTS AND INNER VOICE.

EXPLANATIONS AND DEBUNKING THE MISCONCEPTIONS.

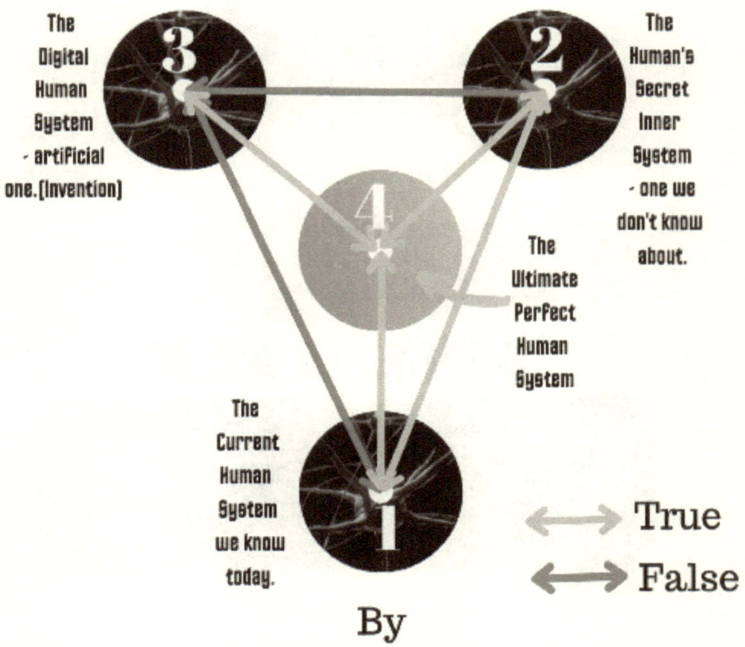

By

David Gomadza

President & Founder
Tomorrow's World Order

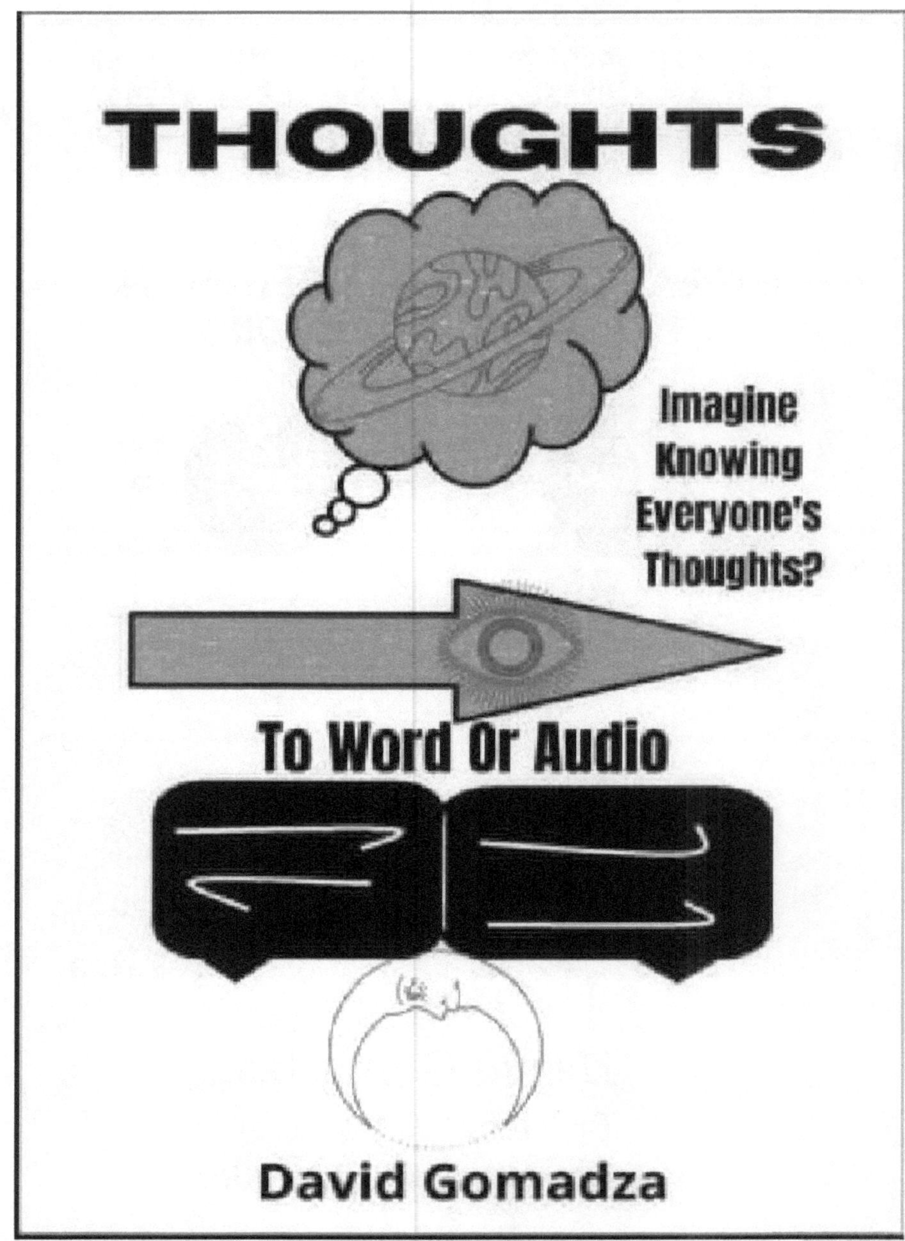
THOUGHTS
Imagine
Knowing
Everyone's
Thoughts?
To Word Or Audio
David Gomadza